# HOMEBIRTH

## Safe & Sacred

Kim Woodard Osterholzer

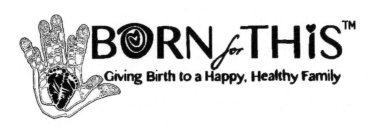

Revised 2020

ISBN-10: 1689254939
ISBN-13: 978-1689254939

COVER PHOTO
Danica Donnelly of *Danica Donnelly Photography*

Also by Kim Woodard Osterholzer

*A Midwife in Amish Country*
*Nourish + Thrive*
*One Little Life at a Time*


Learn more at

KimOsterholzer.com
SafeSacredBirth.com

# CONTENTS

This little book is for the woman who believes she was born to bring her unborn child into the light of day with power, with dignity.

This little book is for the woman
who would accomplish such an inimitable feat
in the tranquility of her own home
if she thought it safe to do so.

This little book, then, my dear sister, is for you.

"Learn to treat this sacred moment of birth
as fragile, as fleeting, as elusive as dawn."

Fredrick Leboyer, MD; *Birth Without Violence* (1)

...

"Imagine if our culture told us birth
was one of the greatest things a woman might ever do.
Imagine if the stories and images we were exposed to
taught us labor is an incredible and transformative experience,
a rite of passage..."

Leonie MacDonald; *Birth Journeys* (2)

...

"A woman in birth is at once
her most powerful and most vulnerable.
Any woman who's birthed unhindered
understands we're stronger than we know."

Marcie Macari; *She Births* (3)

"Things aren't always what they seem;
the first appearance deceives many..."

Plato

# 1

## IF IT IS REALLY RISKIER

*Once upon a time...*

A midwife woke to the jangling of her telephone.

She slipped away from the warm body in her bed, found the clothing she'd draped over the chair beside the dresser, closed the door softly behind her, and crept down the stairs in the dark.

She entered her cozy kitchen and started the kettle to boil, then dialed her assistant's number while gathering her gear.

Soon the woman was easing from her driveway beneath a brilliant wash of glittering stars with a steaming cup of coffee in her hand and a million thoughts tumbling through her head.

As she made her way through the maze of darkish streets

between her and her client's home, her mind drifted back to the first time this family had jangled at her telephone lines.

"Hello, this is Kate!"

"Hi, Kate, my name is Lillian. I got your number from Beth. I'm obviously calling to see about a homebirth with you—but—"

And Lillian surprised Kate by bursting into a flood of tears.

"But I don't really want a homebirth—we just have to have one because we recently switched insurance providers, and now it will cost a lot more to have our baby in the hospital. We looked into birthing at home and feel it's safe enough, so we thought we'd interview with you, if you're willing—"

More tears.

"I'm sorry, I'm just not the homebirthing type. I love my doctor and we had a great birth in the hospital our first time around—though we didn't actually have my doctor at the birth and I didn't especially like the doctor we got—she was short about the pain I was in while she stitched me up afterward. I got a third-degree tear and she said, 'Well, that's what happens when a mom doesn't get an epidural.' But we wanted a natural birth, and we got what we wanted.

"He came fast! No one seemed ready for him to come so fast! My labor was only three hours long. And it was intense! I was screaming and John—that's my husband—he didn't know what to do! The nurse kept yelling for me not to push while the doctor tried to get her gloves on—then suddenly our son was out and in my arms! We were sooo happy! But that tear repair was awful, and then my postpartum was pretty hard—"

Lillian took a deep breath.

"Wow. Sorry! I didn't mean to say all that! I don't even know where it came from!"

"Oh, that's no problem, Lillian," Kate said, "I want to hear your story. I'm glad you enjoyed your hospital birth, and I'm very sorry you feel like you have to have a homebirth now."

Lillian and John met with Kate a few nights later and, despite Lillian's sorrow, the three of them hit it off. Lillian was worried about a few things, though. She'd been diagnosed with a subchorionic hematoma by ultrasound and her doctor said she'd be a little more likely to have her baby too early and possibly even bleed too much when she gave birth.

They discussed the actual measure of increased risk she faced per those issues, the steps she could take during the remainder of her pregnancy to reduce them, and how Kate would handle either complication should one or both manifest.

Lillian and John were satisfied with the meeting. They settled into Kate's care and began preparing for their homebirth.

Kate's thoughts returned to the present as she pulled into Lillian's driveway.

She parked, loaded her shoulders with three big bags of gear, a birth stool, and Lillian's chart, and started for the front door.

. . . . . . .

"I know it's riskier," the man said, "but my wife would really like to have a homebirth this time—"

I smiled. "Okay. Let's start with that."

Those were the opening lines of a recent consultation, and a reflection of what lies behind the polite smiles of most people I meet when they first learn I'm a homebirth midwife.

The idea of homebirth appeals to many on a great many levels, but the commonly-held belief it's extra risky holds most at bay.

And, if it really is riskier, those reservations are far more than reasonable.

Nearly thirty years ago my own young husband, a protectively skeptical police officer, found himself perplexed by the homebirthing hopes and dreams sparkling in my eyes while our first child swam serenely within the waters of my secret places.

Ultimately, we went beyond resolving his assortment of concerns to birthing both of our children at home and getting me through a homebirth midwifery apprenticeship.

Since our early days, I've enjoyed the incomparable privilege of serving homebirthing women as apprentice and then midwife for more than twenty-seven years, welcoming 600 souls as they burst into life, including the souls of our five most delightful grandchildren. Our oldest child has become a homebirth midwife, too.

But—back to our question.

Is homebirth riskier?

The answer to that question is what I hope to shine a bit of light on through the pages of this book.

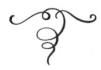

"Experiences have clearly shown an approach
which de-medicalizes birth,
restoring dignity and humanity to the process,
and returning control to the mother,
is also the safest approach."

Michel Odent, MD; *Birth Reborn* (4)

...

"The trick is to be totally non-interventive when things are going well,
and still be ready to act immediately if not."

Anne Frye, CPM; *Holistic Midwifery, Volume II* (5)

...

"A good midwife has a good pair of hands,
and she knows how to sit on them."

Author Unknown

# 2

# HOMEBIRTH

Kate reached the door of Lillian and John's home and let herself in.

Bear, the couple's ancient, oversized black poodle, greeted her with an infectious enthusiasm that belied his years.

Kate smiled and ruffled his ears as she slid her shoes from her feet and her gear from her shoulders.

"Excited about the baby, Buddy?"

His long, pink tongue flicked her cheek while his tail thwacked about at her thighs.

"Yes, yes! I guess you are."

Kate tied her apron around her waist and glanced at the watch on her wrist.

It had only taken her about forty minutes to reach the family from the time they'd called for her to come, and Lillian hadn't noticed but a few contractions prior to that, so Kate supposed they'd have a little while before the baby made his appearance. Still, just in case, Kate pulled her birth tote from its bag to bring along with her doppler, blood pressure monitor, and Lillian's chart when she tip-toed down the hall to Lillian and John's bedroom.

She would have known where to go even if she hadn't already been shown through their home. The familiar sing-song of a woman in labor drew her toward the last door on the left.

Kate paused when she reached it and listened.

"You're doing great, Lillian. I'm so proud of you."

Kate smiled as she tapped lightly on the door.

"Come on in..."


． ． ． ． ． ． ．


A mere 1-2% of Americans give birth to their children beyond hospital doors. (6) I personally believe if the truth about the safety of homebirth was more widely known, that number would rise.

As it is, a pernicious misunderstanding of homebirth safety exists and persists and is perpetuated, I trust unwittingly, by a host of well-meaning medical professionals.

For example, a comparison of home and hospital birthing outcomes was published by a team led by Joseph R. Wax, MD in 2010. It was entitled, "Maternal and Newborn Outcomes in Planned Home Birth vs Planned Hospital Birth: A Meta-analysis." (7) Needless to say, its conclusion that planned homebirth is three times as likely to result in dead babies as planned hospital birth sent the out-of-hospital birthing community reeling.

A closer look at the analysis, however, produced a collective sigh of relief. Not only was it marred by a series of erroneous computations and subject to random inclusions and exclusions of studies, but data was pulled from a number of substandard, contradictory studies, as well as from birth certificate worksheet records where all out-of-hospital births were lumped together for evaluation. That means the study included planned and unplanned births, births attended by skilled practitioners as well as those poorly attended, births completely unattended, and births occurring outside of the hospital purely by accident, rendering the conclusions of the study irrelevant. (8; 9)

Since the publication of this confusing study, several additional studies and analyses of homebirth have been published, confirming its safety. (10; 11; 12; 13; 14; 15) The most recent of these at the time of writing is a systematic review and meta-analysis published by *The Lancet*. Researchers looked at fourteen studies including data from around 500,000 intended homebirths. They found "the risk of perinatal or neonatal mortality was not different when birth was intended at home or in hospital." (14) A common thread running through these and many other studies on this topic is how much less intervention women and their babies experience when women choose to give birth at home.

## Midwifery and Midwifery Training

There are two branches upon the tree that is American midwifery. One branch of that tree is Certified Nurse Midwifery (CNM), a Registered Nurse's graduate degree. The other is traditional or direct-entry midwifery.

Certified Professional Midwifery (CPM) is a limb upon the latter branch. CPMs are direct-entry midwives who've submitted themselves to the scrutiny and standards of a body of fellow midwives, the North American Registry of Midwives (NARM) (16), for the purposes of personal accountability and quality assurance. The route to certification with NARM may include enrollment in a school of midwifery, or may simply employ apprenticeship with a more seasoned CPM. Many midwives are educated via a coupling of routes. (16) In states that register or license their direct-entry midwives, the CPM is generally the criterion. The NARM Bridge Certificate is increasingly required as well. (16)

CPMs are the only birthworkers in the United States trained specifically to attend out-of-hospital birth. Each student must attend a minimum of fifty-five predominantly out-of-hospital births—twenty-five as primary attendants, albeit under direct supervision—in order to secure certification, though many of us attended upwards of one hundred or even two hundred births before receiving our coveted certificates. (16)

## Homebirth Midwifery Statistics

*The Journal of Midwifery* published a study in 2014 called, "Outcomes of Care for 16,924 Planned Home Births in the United States: The Midwives Alliance of North America Statistics Project, 2004 to 2009." (6) It tracked planned homebirths over a span of six years and revealed an impressive array of evidence supporting the practice as plentifully safe for low-risk moms and their babes, as did the study that came before it, "The CPM 2000 Project," published in 2005 and examining 5,418 planned homebirths. (17)

Of the 16,924 women planning to give birth at home, fully 89.1% of them accomplished just that. Of the 11% who were taken to the hospital—mostly for trouble progressing—another 4.5% (for a grand total of 93.6%) were yet able to birth spontaneously, while 1.2% managed instrumentally assisted vaginal births and 5.2% birthed by cesarean section. (6)

Most babies were born in excellent condition with five-minute Apgar scores of seven or greater.

Excluding lethal fetal anomalies, 1.3 in 1000 babies died during their births and 0.76 in 1000 babies died at or shortly after their births. These figures further confirm the safety of homebirth, as the national rates of baby loss are much higher than this. However, because women who birth at home are generally low-risk, and because different studies use different definitions, it's difficult to make exact comparisons. Analysis of the data failed to indicate these babies would have been saved had they been born in the hospital.

Transfers of moms and/or babies to the hospital after birth were rare.

Most babies—86%—were still breastfeeding exclusively by six weeks post birth.

These stellar results were accompanied by a tremendous measure of client satisfaction and were achieved at a fraction of what it typically costs for birth to be accomplished inside the American hospital system.

The safety of homebirth midwifery is greatly enhanced when midwifery and medical systems are well-integrated. While the opportunity for such integration appears to be increasing, it's still rarely available here in the United States. (18)

Such integration is beautifully demonstrated by a study published in the BJOC in 2009 called "Perinatal Mortality and Morbidity in a Nationwide Cohort of 529,688 Low-risk Planned Home and

Hospital Births." (19) The study covered seven years and the entire country of the Netherlands. All births were conducted by midwives with most (60.7%) intended to take place in homes. The mortality and morbidity rates of both mothers and babies were low, with "no significant differences" noted between intended places of birth.

The following statement concludes the study: "This study shows that planning a home birth doesn't increase the risks of perinatal mortality and severe perinatal morbidity among low-risk women, provided the maternity care system facilitates this choice through the availability of well-trained midwives, and through a good transportation and referral system." (19)

## Whom may midwives serve?

Marsden Wagner, perinatologist and perinatal epidemiologist, among others, estimated that 80-85% of women and their babies bear an adequately low burden of risk through pregnancy, birth, and the postpartum period to receive midwifery care either in their homes or at independent birthing centers. (20; 21; 22) Midwifery care has even been presented as a possible solution for improving American birthing outcomes. (18; 22)

## Low-Risk Moms and Babies

I'd like to take a moment to address a point that's often made when comparing midwives and doctors, out-of-hospital births and hospital births.

In the United States, midwives in all settings are said to serve low-risk women, while doctors serve all women. This isn't the case in other countries where midwives are a part of the health care system and serve women regardless of perceived risk status.

But risk really can be something of a perception issue, and it should be understood that steps taken to avoid one risk will often introduce yet another risk or even set of risks. Induction of labor is a good illustration of this. Within health care systems, induction is offered in the hope of reducing the risk of stillbirth, but there isn't always good evidence it does this, and it carries many other risks to women and their babies. This equates far more to an exchange of risk than to an elimination of risk. Therefore, when considering such an exchange, it's essential each potential risk be carefully examined and properly weighed.

For example, medicine considers moms past the age of 35, mothers considered to have a high BMI (or body mass index), mamas who've borne seven or more babies (sometimes fewer), moms whose pregnancies pass 42 or even only 41 weeks gestation, women attempting to give birth after having a baby or babies by cesarean section, moms carrying twins, and mothers carrying breech babies to be moderate to high-risk birthers.

It's certainly true women in these situations have a higher chance of experiencing problems—most especially those carrying breech or twin babies or those desiring to birth vaginally after having birthed by cesarean section—but it's important to recognize these factors are only one element of a woman's health and circumstances. While the presence of these risk factors may indicate a higher chance of a problem on a population level, it doesn't mean all women will have problems. Many midwives are willing to evaluate such birthers on a case-by-case basis. Provided such birthers and their babies present favorably and remain favorable for birth out-of-hospital—yes, by midwifery standards—midwives often will agree to serve them. (5)

Most midwives and doctors consider the worst of birthing risks to be catastrophic events—prolapsed cords, abrupted placentas, ruptured uteri, shoulder dystocias, and breech birth obstructions, to name the top offenders. Catastrophic events tend to arise suddenly and with little warning, and they leave all involved dramatically shaken, especially as mortality and morbidity rates for catastrophic events, wherever they transpire, are higher.

Fortunately, catastrophic events are exceedingly rare occurrences—rare enough to resist the urge to manage all labors and births as though they're very likely to happen, especially in the cases of truly low-risk moms and babes and their reputation for being able to birth, as already indicated, without incidents of any kind.

## The Midwifery Model of Care

The wonderful outcomes enjoyed by the majority of homebirthing families flow from a deeply basic understanding of and trust in the processes of carrying, birthing, and nurturing babies that midwives term "The Midwifery Model of Care." (23)

Midwives understand and trust the carrying, birthing, and nurturing of babies are profoundly sacred and transformative processes and, for all the births a midwife may attend over the course of her career, the birth she's attending at any given moment will never, ever happen again.

Midwives understand and trust the processes of carrying, birthing, and nurturing babies has the power to affect those who experience it in uncountable ways for the duration of their lifetimes.

Midwives understand and trust the carrying, birthing, and nurturing of babies are remarkably normal processes that most commonly occur without incident or the need for intervention.

Midwives understand and trust that because the carrying, birthing, and nurturing of babies are remarkably normal processes, what birthing souls require most is sensitive, respectful attention as the process unfurls.

Midwives also understand that the way people are treated by their health care providers has a direct effect on their outcomes, with the accessory factors of race, sexual orientation, religious belief, income level, size, and age bearing heavily upon the quality of care they're likely to receive. (24; 25; 26; 27; 28; 29; 30)

The word, doula, means to serve.

The word, midwife, means with woman.

While a doula is not a midwife nor a midwife a doula, most midwives in America feel very strongly that the roles of each are inextricably entwined.

Though midwives do indeed possess the knowledge and skills necessary to negotiate the thrills and challenges that arise from time to time in the midst of birthing, since the greater percentage of women are able to give birth to babies spontaneously with a similar ratio of babies arriving vigorous and thriving, most of a midwife's time may simply be spent examining, reassuring, heartening, explaining, soothing, feeding, watering, wiping, tidying, and charting. Midwives do a lot of admiring, too.

Midwives provide continuous, individualized care that acknowledges, promotes, and safeguards the process of childbearing for low-risk moms and babies. Midwives are also adept at recognizing potential issues from afar and circumventing those issues well ahead of their full manifestations. When such prevention proves inadequate, midwives will facilitate the transfer of mom and baby to the hospital, continuing to care for them en-route in order to make sure they arrive in stable condition. In 2019, Canadian researchers looked at the outcomes of babies born to women who planned homebirths but lived more than thirty minutes from a hospital with the capacity to do a cesarean. They found no statistically significant differences in Apgar scores, perinatal mortality, and emergency medical service usage. (31)

The care provided by a midwife is a compilation of her education, skill set, experience, and intuition—a portion of which is medical and calls for the use of medical equipment. But chief among a midwife's competence is her ability to connect with her clients and create a safe space for them to be drawn out, to be heard, to have their experiences validated, and their needs expressed and met. A midwife teaches, encourages, inspires, empowers, and entrains with her clients as she supports and serves them. A midwife's best tools are her ears, her heart, her hands. Midwives individualize the care they provide, allowing the results of their measurements and assessments to be influenced and tempered by the determinations, the beliefs, the hopes, the desires, the histories, and the dreams of the women she's tending.

A midwife's commitment truly is to be with the women she serves—with them creating environments ideal for the carrying, birthing, and nurturing of their babies, then standing sentinel over them and those environs as woman after woman loses herself in consummate metamorphosis.

## A Handful of Specifics

While there are many things unique to what homebirth midwives do to ensure the families in their care enjoy the best possible outcomes, a few of those things are worthy of a closer look.

Elizabeth Davis, Dr. Sara Wickham, Anne Frye, and Ina May Gaskin—to name my favorite few—have written and lectured extensively on the subject of physiologic birth and its many benefits to the blossoming family. Trusting and yielding to the process of growing and birthing and nourishing new life inspires a delicious ebb and flow of hormones that do so much more than simply promote optimal childbearing. When families approach the experience open to immersion in that trust and all that issues from it, the hearts and souls of each involved are primed to coalesce in almost astonishing ways, triggering the integration of the baby, not only into superb physical health, but into a state of emotional and social vigor that will see the nascent being through the duration of his or her lifetime. (32; 33)

The principal pillars I consider this inimitable system to stand upon are the facilitation of undisturbed birth, the preservation of the waters, the optimal clamping and cutting of the cord, the provision of immediate and sustained skin-to-skin contact with mother and dad, and the provision for an uninterrupted hour or two following birth.

## Undisturbed Birth

"In birth, as in making love, privacy is crucial."
—Elizabeth Davis, CPM; *Orgasmic Birth* (32)

33

"The end of pregnancy is as miraculous as its beginning."
—Judith Lothian, RN; "Saying 'No' to Induction" (34)

"Natural labour itself begins slowly for some women, perhaps with the finding of a plug of blood-streaked mucus when they visit the toilet or with the slow and gradual onset of waves of sensation in their wombs during the night. For others natural labour starts more suddenly, perhaps as the waters release with a gush." —Dr. Sara Wickham; *Inducing Labour, Making Informed Decisions* (35)

Making space for undisturbed and gentle birth is central to the excellent outcomes the clients of homebirth midwives regularly experience, and it begins with recognizing the mysterious, miraculous milieu that sparked the genesis of the child so many months before promises also to be the very magic that will bring the child to and through his or her birth.

Novelty. Vulnerability. Love. Respect. Intimacy. Passion. Agony. Ecstasy. Triumph.

Those aspects belonging almost solely to the human experience bloom best in the soil of privacy and, in the context of labor, usher mom and baby and dad into the altered states of mind culminating in such glorious birth the glow of it stands to warm and illumine long after.

I guess you could say the excellent outcomes the clients of homebirth midwives regularly experience begin and end with the mysterious, miraculous milieu that sparked the genesis of the child.

With that in mind, midwives work assiduously with the families they serve to make and preserve spaces conducive to undisturbed, spontaneous birthing.

The family provides the sanctuary the mother would like to birth within, then they fill it with whatever best creates the ambiance desired.

That may include candles, music, essential oils, flowers, a

birthing pool, a stack of warm blankets, a pile of pillows, and most special loved ones.

Sometimes it includes nothing but themselves and all they're most familiar with.

The midwives contribute by endeavoring to support the family as unobtrusively as possible, honoring the environment they've crafted. Using hushed tones and slow movements, they encourage food and drink, and advocate movement and rest and surrender by turns while employing their carefully cultivated powers of observation in order to reduce clinical assessments of vitals and progress to that which is essential—minding the flavor of the family and the rhythm of the labor ever and all the while.

Always working with the design.
Always working with.
Always with.

## Preservation of the Waters

The amniotic sac is a remarkably designed entity that lends itself with near perfection to the endeavor of nourishing and protecting the well-being of the pre-born child.

The determination to preserve the integrity of the amniotic sac is the determination to preserve the protection it provides—protection from infection, protection from umbilical cord compromise, protection from the forces of labor, protection even from the mother's pelvis and musculature.

American homebirth midwives only very rarely rupture amniotic sacs. Most of the time the sacs release on their own as mothers labor, but sometimes babies are born fully enclosed within their waters.

There's hardly a thing more breathtaking than to witness a little life spiraling into the light with her lovely lavender body suspended in a perfect teardrop of her fluids—her turgid, turquoise coil of cord encircled with ribbons of ruby vessels swirling around beside her.

If the waters don't release even when the child comes fully forth, a fingertip may be pressed gently between her rosebud lips till the sac pops. All then that remains is to peel the shimmering swath of tissue from her face as her cries ripple and ring through the room.

## Optimally-Timed Cord Clamping and Cutting

Speaking of the turgid, turquoise coil of cord with its ribbons of ruby vessels, George Malcolm Morley, MB, ChB, FACOG composed a stunning article in 2003 called, "Neonatal Resuscitation: Life that Failed," in which he describes the importance of leaving the newborn baby's lifeline unclamped and uncut during and after his or her birth. (36)

Dr. Morley reminds us the unborn child grows within his mother's womb in a sub-oxygenated state and therefore bursts forth into daylight, as we've already mentioned, a lovely shade of purple. The first infilling of his wee lungs sends a glorious wash of pink the length and breadth of his untouched skin while the surges of warm blood flowing to him from his placenta aids the expansion of those lungs, flushing and "activating" a more mature functioning of the rest of his little organs. (36)

Dr. Morley describes this process as that of "natural resuscitation," and admonishes its dependence on the "copious perfusion" provided by the bolus of placental blood coursing to the baby

36

in great waves following his birth. This "transfusion" is "regulated and terminated reflexively by the child and results in a blood volume optimal for survival." (36)

"Immediate cord clamping," the doctor goes on to say, "produces major deviations from natural resuscitation: placental oxygenation, placental acidosis regulation, placental glucose supply, and placental transfusion are all abruptly aborted and the child is subjected to a period of complete asphyxiation until the lungs (begin to) function… The immediately clamped newborn has, in effect, been subjected to a massive hemorrhage, losing up to 50% of its blood volume."

He goes further to state that when a child is balancing along the knife-edge of stability through or upon his birth—something providers may or may not be fully cognizant of—immediate cord clamping has the power to "seal its fate."

A researcher Dr. Morley cites in his article, T. Peltonen, states, "On the basis of these observations, it would seem that the closing of the umbilical circulation before aeration of the lungs has taken place is a highly unphysiologic measure which should thus be avoided. Although the normal infant survives… under certain unfavorable conditions, the consequences may be fatal." (36)

There are a number of short and long-term benefits to keeping the umbilical cord intact including fewer babies requiring resuscitation, fewer babies requiring neonatal intensive care, fewer babies suffering inadequate hemoglobin levels through the first year of life and, in turn, fewer children suffering learning and behavior issues. (36; 37)

Another benefit optimal cord clamping and cutting provides—with the term, "optimal," being one Dr. Nadine Edwards and Dr. Sara Wickham suggest as possibly more appropriate than the term, "delayed" (37)

—dovetails with our next point of discussion. Babies whose cords are left alone are far more likely to be allowed hours to bask naked and unafraid upon their mothers' warm, bare breasts following their births.

Most midwives recognize the value of preserving the vital connection between babies and their placentas, and work industriously to honor it. Many also realize all that clamping and cutting cords once they're "finished pulsing" does is disrupt the unrepeatable, irreplaceable process of bonding and integration.

## Immediate and Sustained Skin-to-Skin Contact

Immediate and sustained skin-to-skin contact after birth is all about the stabilization of newborn babies and the promotion of bonding and integration.

Nils Bergman, MD and his wife, Jill, developed what the world has come to know as Kangaroo Care. (38; 39; 40; 41; 42)

Kangaroo Care embodies the endeavor to expediate the stabilization of newborn babies as they transition to life outside the womb via the body of their very own mothers. When naked babies are placed wet and squirming on the naked breasts of their mothers, the nervous systems of each instantly begin a synchronistic dance that rapidly equilibrates babies' temperatures, pulses, blood pressures, and blood glucose levels.

Initially, Kangaroo Care was employed on behalf of premature babies born in countries without access to advanced care systems, but it didn't take long for the Bergmans to realize continuous time skin-to-skin with mothers—and dads, actually—is a fundamental requirement of all babies.

Recognition of the virtual imperative of immediate and

sustained skin-to-skin connection between mother and babe is ubiquitous among homebirth midwives and comprises, in concert with the preservation of the umbilical cord, one of the primary reasons so very few homeborn babies require extensive resuscitative efforts, much less transfer to hospital neonatal intensive care units. (38; 39; 40; 41; 42)

## An Uninterrupted Hour or Two Following Birth

"Sensations fire and wire the brain. During breastfeeding all the senses work together to make pathways and circuits into networks. So, taste and smell, as well as sight and sound and warmth and touch and pressure and balance and movement are integrated." —Jill Bergman, Doula; "For Full Term Babies" (39)

This marvelous system of integration creates what the Bergmans call "secure attachment" and engenders life-long physical, emotional, and social health. (38; 39; 40; 41; 42)

Skin-to-skin communion also lends itself to an infant's increasing intelligence and the development of a mother's protective instincts.

"The number of hours of skin-to-skin contact baby receives in the first day of life will determine his mother's sensitivity to his cognitive development and emotional security even a year later. This also predicts the attachment relationship and social intelligence." —Jill Bergman, Doula; "The Importance of Skin-to-Skin Contact for Every Newborn" (40)

This period of time is vital. It's far more than eating, as there's only a teaspoon or so of colostrum in a newly-birthed mother's breasts. The baby is soothing himself after all the sudden changes caused by his birth and, even more importantly, he's bonding indelibly with his family.

This quiet spell in the bed is a wonderful time for a family to enjoy a meal together while admiring the baby and marveling over his birth. In the meantime, the midwife will be puttering about nearby, tidying things up, putting things away, filling out paperwork, checking on the firmness of the birthing mom's uterus and the quantity of her blood flow, and assessing the mother's perineum for tears until the family indicates the baby's through nursing and ready to be examined.

Once the midwife has examined the baby and displayed his placenta to his parents, the baby will enjoy a spell of skin-on-skin with his dad while the midwife sees mom to the toilet and shower and back. Then she'll reassess mom's uterus and blood flow, evaluate her vitals, and tuck the trio into bed. At the third to fourth hour after the birth of the baby—as long as both are doing well—the midwife will go on home. By this time, most moms and babies—and very oftentimes dads—will be sleeping peacefully, so the midwife simply locks the door and pulls it closed behind her.

## What to Expect When Tended by a Midwife Continuity of Care

Chief among the many splendid benefits enjoyed while enveloped in the care of American homebirth midwives is the opportunity afforded the mother-baby dyad to be tended before, during, and after birth by a single provider.

When one person is gathering and assessing vitals, readings, reports, and measurements, that one person becomes intimately acquainted with her charges, and is thereby uniquely poised to detect and interpret even the most subtle of shifts. Then also her subsequent recommendations will be consistent, and any necessary sharing or transferring of care with or to other providers will be accomplished more effectively and efficiently.

## Conscientious Preventative Care

Accented by this stand-alone system of consistent care is the midwife's ability to assist those they serve as they work to achieve the best states of health and well-being possible in order to experience the pregnancy, labor, birth, new parenting, and season of recovery they hope for.

An expectant woman's midwife will work with her to customize a plan for getting great rest, mindful exercise, top-notch nutrition and hydration, and to achieve an ideal state of heart and soul—all positioning the mother-to-be to embrace and enjoy what stands to be one of her life's grandest catalysts for transformation.

## Prenatal Care

After gaining assurance families are making fully informed decisions to experience pregnancy, birth, and postpartum in the home setting, midwives take the plunge with them into prenatal care. The care journey described in this and the following sections is typical for American midwives, but many variations may be experienced, both in the United States and between the United States and elsewhere.

From the 10th or 12th week of pregnancy through the 28th week, midwives and their clients meet for visits once every four weeks.

From the 28th week through the 36th week, they meet every other week. Then, from the 36th week till the birth of the baby, meetings are kept weekly.

The visits usually last an hour or two, though the first visit may take a bit longer as, besides making a first physical assessment, portions of it will be spent filling out and signing policy papers, reviewing health history forms, and collecting blood samples for laboratory work-ups.

The 28th and 36th week visits are often longer, too, as samples are gathered for second rounds of lab work and additional sets of paperwork are filled out and signed. Usually the 36th week meetings are home visits where supplies and the spots in houses where families plan to birth may be inspected. Many midwives offer a short childbirth education class to first-time parents at the 36th week as well.

Midwife visits include assessments of urine for leukocytes, blood, protein, nitrites, ketones, and glucose, at the least. Weights, blood pressures, fundal heights, estimations of fetal sizes, fetal heart tone rates and variabilities, and positions and presentations of babies and how they relate with the pelves of their mothers are measured. A great many questions are asked about how often babies move, how active uteri are, what vaginal secretions are like, how diets and appetites are, how moms are sleeping, whether moms are exercising, if moms have sprouted any varicosities, and how easy it is for mamas to empty their bladders and evacuate their colons. Other questions are asked such as whether moms are experiencing swelling, headaches, dizziness, visual disturbances, or any pains in their heads, chests, abdomens, legs, or elsewhere.

Time is spent then exploring how women are doing emotionally and psychologically, and spread throughout the visit are considerations of women's questions and concerns, as well as discussions regarding drink, food, supplements, exercise, and the pursuit of complimentary therapies such as chiropractic care, physical therapy, massage, acupuncture, and mental health therapists.

All along the way midwives provide a variety of reading and viewing materials, as well as abundant time to discuss what expectant mamas have weighing on their minds or in their hearts.

## Birth Care

Exactly when a midwife heads out to attend a woman's birth depends on which of her babies she's expecting.

If she's a first-time mom or a first-time vaginal birther, that's usually when her contractions are coming every three to five minutes, lasting sixty seconds or so, and have been following such a pattern for about an hour.

If a woman's had a baby vaginally before, midwives usually make their start when contractions are coming every eight to ten minutes, lasting forty-five to sixty seconds, and have been doing so for an hour.

Of course, a midwife just never can predict how things will go with a woman, regardless how many babies she's had or hasn't had. Depending on what the midwife finds when she arrives, she may wind up going back home for a while, but when a woman calls for her midwife to come see her in her labor, she responds.

The first thing a midwife does when she arrives is take a reading of both the mom's and the baby's vitals—chiefly, maternal blood pressure and pulse and fetal heart tones—the latter usually through a contraction. She assesses the woman's pattern of contractions, then, especially if the woman is a first-timer, the midwife may ask to check her cervical effacement and dilation, to assess the station of the baby, and to confirm that the presenting part of the baby really and truly is its head.

The midwife then sets up her gear and the woman's supplies and tucks herself away in some corner of her house—within ear-shot—to get started on the paperwork.

Usually the midwife isn't too needed until the woman feels like she could push. By and large moms and dads work beautifully together through their labors and births—very much the way they work together through the courses of their lives.

Every half hour to hour the midwife assesses the baby's heart tones for rate and variability. She also makes sure the woman is eating and drinking, resting if possible, peeing often, handling her contractions well, and moving along about as expected. Should she not move along as expected, the midwife explores why, as well as what may be done to alter that, if altering that would be appropriate.

When the mother begins to feel like pushing, the midwife will encourage her to let her body do the bulk of the work without adding too much oomph to its efforts in order to keep the process gentle for both her baby and for her unfurling tissues. Midwives keep a close eye on the baby as he makes his way along his warm, dark path, checking the rhythm of his heart every five to ten minutes while the woman breathes, breathes, breathes him steadily toward the light.

And at last! With a rush of laughter and spray of tears, he slips into his father's or his mother's hands! Though sometimes he slips into the hands of his midwife.

The midwife spends the next three to four hours receiving the placenta, checking and re-checking the pair's vitals, assessing the condition of the woman's uterus and blood flow, examining and repairing her tissues as necessary, assisting with nursing, tidying up messes, fetching food and drink, examining the baby from head to toe, helping the mother toilet and bathe, and finishing off the paperwork. Midwives are careful to depart only when the mother and baby are stable and all tasks are completed.

# Postpartum Care

As with prenatal visits, typical postpartum visits provided by American homebirth midwives last from one to two hours, with second visits taking a bit longer to allow for collections of blood samples for the Newborn Screen. Midwives generally visit newly-birthed families between twenty-four and thirty-six hours, at the fourth to sixth days, at the tenth to fourteenth days, then at six weeks post-birth, providing all goes well.

Any time additional visits are needed—be they prenatal or postpartum—they're readily provided.

The first postpartum visit is the most thorough. Assessment of the baby's pulse and respiratory rates are made, his heart and lungs sounds are carefully assessed, his oxygen saturation levels are measured, his temperature is taken, his color is examined, his navel and cord stump explored, and he's hoisted to the sky for a weight check. The midwife then turns her attention to the mother and takes a reading of her blood pressure and pulse, makes a survey of her uterus and an assessment of her blood flow and afterpains, and checks on how well her hinder parts are healing. Throughout the visit the state of the breastfeeding relationship and the condition of the mother's breasts are discussed, as well as how both mother and baby are sleeping and eliminating, and how well the mother is eating and drinking and feeling emotionally and psychologically.

The following visits are similar, with discussions expanding to include the resumption of the mother's activities. At the six-week visit the midwife examines the mother's core and pelvic floor musculature and instructs her as to the furtherance of its rejuvenation. The midwife also offers the mother a thorough well-woman exam at this visit, including a pap test.

Many midwives offer twelve-week visits as well.

## Transportation to the Hospital

Midwives invest one hundred percent of their heart, knowledge, intuition, skill, and sweat in keeping the families they serve at home as long as there truly is hope for a good, safe birth there, and their statistics attest to their notable ability to do so.

Still, midwives begin to consider transport a while before it's vitally necessary to transport. The idea is for it never to be vitally necessary to transport.

Midwives work hard to discern through the mists of exhaustion, hope, and dread when the goal of birthing safely at home has slipped beyond likelihood, and to come to grips with that understanding before the only options remaining are to transport the mother and/or baby to the hospital by ambulance and/or to require emergency treatment upon arrival there. Midwives also work hard to keep the families they serve a well-informed and active part of the decision-making process.

If a midwife's presence isn't required to keep mom and/or baby stable and/or if the baby's birth isn't imminent, everyone usually drives to the hospital in their own vehicles. If her presence is required to keep mom and/or baby stable and/or the baby's birth is imminent, she'll ride with the mother and/or baby with her gear at the ready. Those qualifiers also determine which hospital is utilized. If time allows, the group heads for the hospital of preference. If time presses, the nearest hospital is the unquestioned destination.

The midwife does her best to phone ahead to the hospital to let them know they're on the way, how to prepare, and, if appropriate to the situation, to request a member of the labor and delivery staff to be on hand at the door upon their arrival.

The first order of business upon arrival is an assessment of the mom and/or baby. The midwife passes the family's charts off to the staff as the way forward is determined. At that time, providing the state of the mom and/or baby allows for discussions of such things, the family's specific concerns and desires will be voiced.

When a midwife takes a family to the hospital, it's because they need something she can't provide. That doesn't mean the family must automatically agree to all the hospital routinely provides the hosts of folks they take care of. Often, transferred families are able to enjoy many of the things they'd looked forward to at home, especially mother or father-assisted birth, optimal cord clamping and cutting, and immediate and sustained skin-to-skin contact with their newborn.

Midwives stay at the hospital until the baby's born, the nursing relationship is well-established, and the mom and dad are ready— physically and psychologically—for her to leave.

Midwives still generally come visit the new family between twenty-four and thirty-six hours postpartum wherever they are and, once they're back snug in their home, resume regular midwifery care. Post-transfer postpartum care is usually a little more involved as everyone will need to process what happened.

# In Case of Emergency—
## Training, Skills, Equipment, Plans

The efficacy of a homebirth midwife isn't solely ensconced within her expertise in facilitating the facets of physiologic birth, but also within her rigorous training, finely-honed skills, specialized equipment, and carefully crafted contingency plans designed to mitigate the full spectrum of complications and emergencies possible during childbirth.

Homebirth midwives are educated and trained to know and oversee normal physiologic pregnancy, labor, birth, post-birth recovery, and well-woman care. The hand-in-glove component to this education and training is simple. If what a midwife witnesses doesn't fall within the range of normal and she's unable to shepherd mother and baby back within the realm of normal, she'll move to secure appropriate medical care.

Thankfully, often when a measure of medical intervention is called for, midwives are still able to provide an adequate measure of intervention, literally "in house."

When external medical attention must be secured, most times the demand is non-emergent. However, homebirth midwives are trained and equipped in the management of immediate threats while in transit ranging from gestational hypertensions or preeclampsias; placental abruptions or disruptions; uterine ruptures; labor dystocias; any manner of destabilized vitals, be they maternal or neonatal; any malpositions or malpresentations; cord prolapses or other cord issues; shoulder dystocias; any maternal and/or neonatal cardiopulmonary issues; postpartum hemorrhages and/or placental expulsion issues; infant malformations; as well as any measure of maternal and/or neonatal birth injuries.

Midwives have access to laboratories and to ultrasound technology. Midwives possess a vast array of equipment for assessing and monitoring both maternal and neonatal well-being, as well as for conducting resuscitations, halting hemorrhages, and repairing tears.

As stated before, there's ample evidence to show that, as long it's possible to reach a hospital where a cesarean section may be performed, should cesarean be deemed necessary, home is a safe place to give birth. (6; 11; 13; 14)

And, again, research shows this is still the case when women live more than thirty minutes from the hospital. (31)

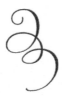

"The physician must…
have two special objects in view with regard to disease,
namely, to do good or to do no harm."

Hippocrates, *Of the Epidemics*

...

"I will follow that system of regimen which,
according to my ability and judgment, I consider for the
benefit of my patients, and abstain from whatever
is deleterious and mischievous."

Hippocrates, *The Hippocratic Oath*

...

"I had an expert midwife who kept meticulous records
of her outcomes. I've never seen an obstetrician at the
first prenatal visit hand over their complete list of how many
thousands of births they'd done, what their overall C-section
rate was, how many complications they had, and what the
complications were. My midwife did that for me and I felt
incredibly safe in her hands. Her statistics were far better
than any of the OBs I'd ever met, or even my own."

Jennifer Lang, OB/GYN, "What if Homebirth is Actually
SAFER than Hospital Birth?" (43)

"My past experiences as a practitioner
had already led me to believe that time and patience
are the most useful of allies, and that active intervention
should be used only sparingly and in special cases."

Michel Odent, MD; *Birth Reborn* (4)

...

"It's therefore understandable that pregnancy
and the birth of a child should have been invested
with special value, as witnessed by the customs, ceremonials,
rituals, and other practices with which these events
are associated in all societies...
A hospital is a splendid place, but it's not, in my view,
a place in which the most beautiful celebration in the history
of a family, the welcoming of a new member into it,
should occur. That event should be celebrated where
it belongs, in the bosom of the family, in the home...
The family is the basis of society. As the family is,
so is the society... (may we find) the safe harbor of
happily born children in happy families where everyone
is given the opportunity to inherit his birthright ...
without the obfuscating and damaging effects
of an outmoded ... traditional obstetrics."

Ashley Montagu, Ph.D.; from the foreword to

Dr. Bradley's *Husband-Coached Childbirth* (44)

# 3

# HOSPITAL BIRTH

Kate eased the door open and slipped inside.

Lillian and John stood together beside the bed, clinging to one another and swaying in time to the profound powers of labor—Lillian breathing, John whispering words of encouragement—riding the awe-inspiring surf as one, just as they'd ridden the whitecaps of passion that had sparked their child into existence ten moons before.

Kate set her tote on a dresser top, then perched on the bed near the pair with her doppler and blood pressure monitor in her lap.

As the wave of sensation that engulfed them crested and began to ebb, Lillian shook her head at Kate and said, "I hope this isn't a false alarm!"

Kate laughed as she squeezed a blob of gel onto the probe of her doppler.

"It isn't."

"How can you tell?"

"I can tell."

John smiled and Lillian straightened a bit to rub the small of her back.

"Right there?" John asked, slipping one of his hands over the place she was trying to reach.

"Yes, right there—only harder. Harder, John. Ahhh—that's it."

"Would you mind if I listened to the baby a minute or two, Lillian?" Kate asked.

Lillian drew her tee-shirt up to expose the broad, round globe of her belly and it made Kate think of all the similar orbs laboring in other places to bring other littles lives earthside.

A noise of static ensued as Kate slid the probe around the left side of Lillian's belly until the reassuring ca-click, ca-click, ca-click issued forth.

Kate looked at her watch and began to count as the red second hand swept its face. "One-forty... one-thirties..."

Ca-click, ca-click, ca-click, ca-click....

"Does he sound okay?" Lillian asked.

"He does, indeed."

Ca-click, ca-click.

"I love that sound," Lillian said.

John said, "So do I," as he rubbed Lillian's back in slow, smooth circles.

"So do I," Kate said and she continued her counting.

Lillian drew a deep breath. "Here comes another one."

"Mind if I listen through it?"

Lillian nodded as she began to breathe and sway her hips. John moved his hand to the rhythm of her swaying and Kate moved with the two just enough to keep the pattering of the baby's heart tones in their ears.

Seventy seconds passed and Lillian took a deep, deep breath.

"Okay. It's going away."

Kate listened another half minute before switching the doppler off. She wiped the glistening gel from Lillian's taut skin and said, "Strong and steady. Your baby's not minding labor one bit."

Kate took Lillian's blood pressure then. "119/72. Good."

She stood up.

"What should we do?" Lillian asked.

"I'd say you should do just what you're doing. It seems to be working."

Lillian nodded again, ran her hands round and round over her yet-exposed belly, and took a deep breath, signaling the start of another wave of sensation.

"It seems to be working perfectly."

Lillian smiled and began to rock her hips like a ship on the seas, and John rubbed and rubbed and rubbed her back as he brushed a kiss against her ear.

． ． ． ． ． ． ．

I'd like to begin this section with a heartfelt acknowledgment.

Every last birth worker on the face of the earth, from obstetrician to midwife, from nurse to doula, from pediatrician to respiratory therapist, intends for you and your baby to survive the process.

We breathe when you breathe, we ache when you ache, we push when you push, and we rejoice when you rejoice.

When you ride the line between life and death, a scarcely imaginable quantity of adrenaline surges through our veins, and we spring into thoroughly rehearsed action.

And when our best efforts to snatch you or your little one to safety fail, your cries of anguish pierce the very deepest points of our souls where they will forever reverberate.

I know.

I've been there, and I've been there with doctors, with nurses, and with other midwives.

I've been there, too, with EMTs and paramedics, with firefighters and police officers, with social workers and coroners and morticians.

Yes.

Everlasting reverberation.

Everlasting.

Though I very sincerely believe what I just wrote, the surprising fact is, despite spending more on mother-baby care than does any other developed nation in the world, (45) according to Harvard University's Maternal Health Task Force and The Kaiser Family Foundation's Health System Tracker, the United States actually also loses and damages more mothers and more babies through the multifaceted process of birth than does any other developed nation in the world. (45; 46; 47; 48) The numbers of American mothers and babies of color perish at alarmingly higher rates than Caucasian mothers and babies—even three to four times higher (26; 30; 45)—and the rate we're losing mothers of all colors is actually on the rise. (45; 46; 47) Dr. Mary-Ann Etiebet, executive director of Merck for Mothers, estimates 60% of these deaths are preventable. (46)

How can this be?

"I looked at people from a narrow medical perspective. I shared the conventional view of childbirth as a 'medical problem' requiring technical 'solutions.'" —Michel Odent, MD; *Birth Reborn* (4)

"Putting yourself in the hands of a high-tech doctor and a high-tech hospital doesn't guarantee you the safest birth... Remember, birth is not an illness." —Marsden Wagner, Perinatologist, Perinatal Epidemiologist, "Technology in Birth: First Do No Harm" (21)

## *The Medical Model of Care in America*

The model of care in American medicine appears to be a principal factor in this regrettable state of affairs (20; 21)—and it just even actually has to be as fully 98-99% of American births occur in American hospitals. (6)

Though overflowing with sincerely good intentions, this model tends to view the bearing of children, stated so succinctly by Dr. Odent in the quote opening this section, as "a 'medical problem' requiring technical 'solutions.'" (4)

It's easy to see, as described by perinatologist and perinatal epidemiologist, Marsden Wagner, how such a view might generate the idea a provider's role is to "deliver" babies rather than simply provide watchful support as women actively give birth. It's also easy to see how this perspective might inadvertently engender the use and even over-use of interventions, with each intervention leading to additional interventions in a seemingly never-ending slide toward the epitome of birth interventions, the cesarean section. (20; 21)

Approximately 32% of American births are accomplished by cesarean section (49), a rate considered too high by the American College of Obstetricians and Gynecologists, the Society for Maternal-Fetal

59

Medicine, and the World Health Organization. (50; 51) Dr. Neel Shah, professor of obstetrics at Harvard Medical School, considers the cesarean section rate in the United States more than half as high as it ought to be. (46) The World Health Organization recommends the cesarean section rate be closer to 10-15%, though more recent examinations of the data argue that this is too low and suggest a rate of up to 19% may be optimal. (50) These figures don't tell the whole story though, as women whose outcomes are considered in the assessment of these percentages have received medicalized care. We know that caseload midwifery care leads to equally good perinatal outcomes with far lower intervention rates, (6; 52) so it may be, if more women had access to midwifery care, lower cesarean rates would be optimal.

Naturally, cesarean section isn't the only factor contributing to our bleak national maternal and neonatal rating. The Centers for Disease Control and Prevention has listed other factors such as increased maternal age, obesity, and a miscellany of chronic medical conditions as possible contributors. (53)

Those possible contributors certainly merit investigation, but this book isn't intended to be an exhaustive piece of work.

To follow the line of thought I've begun to draw regarding the standard medical view of birth in America and the way that view is disposed to direct the care of American mothers and babies, cesarean section, coupled with both the interventions that funnel mothers and babies more rapidly toward cesarean section and the interventions those interventions, as well as cesarean section birth itself, inspires in their wake are the focus of this chapter.

# *If It Ain't Broke...*

If I were to hazard a guess, I'd suppose nearly every grandfather we've met has at one time or other hooked his thumbs through his belt loops, winked, and said, "Well, now, if it ain't broke, don't fix it."

When a birth goes awry, or maybe really doesn't go at all, intervention is essential and, at those times, we're abundantly thankful for it. But what we're talking about here is the 80-85% of mothers who are low-risk and well-suited for care by midwives (20; 21; 22; 52) and their unparalleled ability to give birth to their healthy babies in astounding displays of courage, strength, and sheer joy when properly supported.

The tragedy of American birthing is the ostensible inability of our medical model of care to understand and trust that the carrying, birthing, and nurturing of babies are profoundly sacred and transformative processes, and that they possess the potential to affect those who experience them in uncountable ways for the duration of their lifetimes. Because these remarkably normal processes most commonly occur without incident or the need for intervention when properly supported, what birthing souls require most is sensitive, respectful attention as these processes unfold. Therefore, intervention is far too commonplace. (20; 21)

Again, according to Dr. Marsden Wagner, as well as to the aforementioned Dr. George Morley and Dr. Nils Bergman, the more common of commonplace interventions are as follows: induction and augmentation of labors, medicated labors, instrumentally assisted births, cesarean sections, immediate cord clamping and cutting, and separation of mothers from babies. (20; 21; 36; 38; 39; 40; 41; 42)

Each of these interventions carry substantial risk to both moms and babies, as evidenced by many of the studies cited in this book, as well as a greater chance of additional intervention down the line, sometimes required to counteract the effects of the first intervention. (49; 54; 55) For example, induced labor is more painful than spontaneous labor, involving powerful medications with significant potential side effects. It therefore requires more careful monitoring, restricting women's abilities to move and draw upon the power of their own bodies as well as gravity. For all of these reasons, fetal distress, a tired mother, and an operative birth are more likely when labor is induced. (35)

Below is a list of what, in my opinion, are the direst risks associated with the more common interventions. I won't describe the mechanics of the interventions at this time, as that information is easily found other places. Nor will I describe their benefits as that information literally abounds, as demonstrated by their fantastically widespread utilization.

Which is rather the point.

"Between 50 and 80% of births in most American hospitals involve one or more surgical procedures... Those procedures include drugs to start or speed up labor, episiotomy... placing forceps or a vacuum extractor on the baby's head to pull the baby out... and cesarean section to cut the baby out. In reality, any of these surgical procedures is necessary in no more than 20% of all births." —Marsden Wagner, Perinatologist, Perinatal Epidemiologist, "Technology in Birth: First Do No Harm" (21)

## Induction and Augmentation of Labor

An induction of labor is a serious intervention and, considering

62

so many women would be able to give birth spontaneously if provided adequate support and opportunity to do so, should only be contemplated when the risk of allowing pregnancy to continue truly outweighs the benefits. (20; 21; 35; 56; 57)

An induction of labor presents the following risks: an increased risk of giving birth to a late-preterm baby with ensuing complications; an increased risk of experiencing uterine overstimulation with ensuing complications including destabilizing the baby and rupturing the uterus; an increased risk of experiencing an extra painful labor, an increased need for a medicated labor with ensuing complications; and an increased risk of requiring a cesarean section with ensuing complications. (20; 21; 56; 57)

An augmentation of labor presents essentially the same risks as an induction of labor, though an augmentation is less likely to produce a late-preterm baby. Both induction and augmentation generally involve the use of synthetic Pitocin, and the use of this carries myriad risks to mother and baby. (58) As well as the physical risks, synthetic oxytocin blocks the mother's release of natural oxytocin. As synthetic oxytocin doesn't cross the blood-brain barrier, (59) she and her baby will lack all of the advantages of natural oxytocin. As Dr. Sara Wickham states, "Oxytocin enhances wellbeing, reduces stress and anxiety, and has many beneficial effects relating to pain relief, motherbaby interaction, and other aspects of birth." (60)

In addition, an induction or augmentation of labor requires continuous electronic fetal monitoring which also increases the risk of requiring a cesarean section. (35; 56)

An induction or augmentation of labor is also commonly accompanied by artificial rupture of the membranes and additional cervical examinations which increases the risk of acquiring an intrapartum infection with ensuing complications. (35; 56)

For more information about induction of labor, see Dr. Sara Wickham's book, *Inducing Labour: Making Informed Decisions*.

## Medicated Labor

Medicating a labor has more unsavory effects than most people realize and, considering so many women would be able to give birth spontaneously if provided adequate support and opportunity to do so, should only be contemplated when the risk of experiencing labor unmedicated truly outweigh the benefits. (56; 58; 61)

Medicating a labor presents the following risks: an increased risk of destabilizing the baby with ensuing complications, an increased risk of reducing the efficiency of labor with ensuing complication, an increased risk of requiring an augmentation of labor with ensuing complications, an increased risk of requiring an instrumentally assisted birth with ensuing complications, and an increased risk of requiring a cesarean section with ensuing complications. (56; 58; 61)

## Instrumentally Assisted Birth

An instrumentally assisted birth via forceps or a vacuum extractor also has potentially serious consequences. Again, considering so many women would be able to give birth spontaneously if provided adequate support and opportunity to do so, many experts suggest they should only be contemplated when the risk of birthing unassisted by instruments truly outweighs the benefits. (54; 56; 62)

Instrumentally assisted birth presents the following risks: an increased risk of damaging the baby with ensuing complications; an increased risk of damaging the mother with ensuing complications; and an increased risk of experiencing a shoulder dystocia. (54; 56; 62)

## *Cesarean Section*

"Caesarean section is justified only when benefits outweigh harms." —BMJ: British Medical Journal (63)

Cesarean section is major abdominal surgery and carries many risks. If we lived in a culture where more women received adequate support and opportunity to birth spontaneously, far fewer women would suffer from the short and long-term consequences of this surgery. Delivery by cesarean section should only be considered when the risks of birthing vaginally truly outweigh the benefits.

A cesarean section presents the following risks to mothers: an increased risk of experiencing a postpartum hemorrhage; an increased risk of requiring a blood transfusion; an increased risk of requiring a secondary surgery to remove the uterus; an increased risk of requiring ventilation and temporary tracheostomy; an increased risk of acquiring an infection; an increased risk of forming blood clots; an increased risk of experiencing an amniotic fluid embolism; an increased risk of requiring readmission to the hospital; an increased risk of experiencing difficulties with subsequent pregnancies and births; and an increased risk of death. (47; 43; 45; 46; 47; 49; 50; 51)

Cesarean section presents the following risks to babies: an increased risk of experiencing respiratory distress requiring resuscitation; an increased risk of being admitted to a neonatal intensive care unit; an increased risk of experiencing immediate cord clamping and cutting; an increased risk of experiencing separation from the mother; an increased risk of experiencing difficulties bonding and breastfeeding; a disruption of the microbiome with an increased risk of experiencing subsequent health challenges; and, most notably for cephalic or head-down babies, an increased risk of death. (47; 43; 45; 46; 47; 49; 50; 51; 64)

## Immediate Cord Clamping and Cutting

"Placental function was the only resuscitative option available (prior to modern methods of resuscitation) and its preservation was of obvious value. Destruction of the infant's only functioning life support system was clearly understood to be injurious, not only for the child, but for the physician's reputation. Destruction of physiology invariably produces pathology... Amputation of a functioning placenta and the blood volume contained in it is an obviously injurious procedure." —George Malcolm Morley, MD, "Neonatal Resuscitation: Life that Failed" (36)

Immediate cord clamping and its ensuing complications is still very common in American hospitals, although a growing number of providers are willing to "wait a minute or two" before clamping and cutting cords, and a few are willing to wait a bit longer. The risks are described in detail in the previous chapter. (36; 37)

## Separation of Mother from Baby

"Separation of the newborn baby from the mother is the primary cause of stress... This often causes a cascade of problems and complications requiring ever more intervention from the neonatal health system. Most of this could be avoided by the mind-blowingly simple practice of putting every newborn baby naked onto Mum's bare chest, drying him, and covering both of them. All of the observations and tests can be done while leaving the newborn in his SAFE place." —Jill

Bergman, Doula; "The Importance of Skin-to-Skin Contact for Every Newborn" (40)

"The very best environment for a baby to grow and thrive is the mother's body... Nowadays we're bringing up children in a manner which is essentially pathological." —Nils Bergman, MD; "Kangaroo Mother Care" (40)

Again, though an increasing number of hospitals advertise the promotion of immediate skin-to-skin contact and rooming-in for the mothers and babies they deliver, it's still fairly common for pairs to be separated after birth, especially when almost any measure of resuscitation of the baby is required.

Even when a baby is actually placed directly on his mother, it's commonly over a blanket which is then used to rub the baby dry with vigor. Often almost simultaneously the child is suctioned, the cord is clamped and cut, a complete set of vitals is taken, and a hat is placed on his head. All of these tasks compose a grievous compilation of disruptions (38; 39; 41; 42) to what should be —remember, 80-85% of the time—the glorious moments following birth. They're moments most certainly irretrievable.

The effect of these disruptions is an impaired ability for mother and baby to connect and, subsequently, an increasingly stressed baby. Concern over the stressed baby, instead of signaling the well-meaning team to take a step back and give the two some space, inspires the team to whisk the baby across the room for monitoring. This separation, coupled with all the stressors that have already been unwittingly levied against the tiny life, then produces the very instability the team had hoped to avoid, and the baby is sent to the neonatal intensive care unit. (38; 39; 41; 42)

## *Perception of Experience*

When women attempt to describe almost any degree of the dissatisfaction they feel regarding their hospital birth experiences, they're often admonished and even shamed. After all, they "just ought to be thankful they have a healthy baby," right?

And yet, who do we suppose among those souls isn't thankful for their healthy baby?

The truth is the fact they dare raise the subject at all, despite the healthy baby nestled in their arms, reveals there's much, much more women hope to experience when they give birth than mere survival.

I've chosen to close this chapter with the words of one of my favorite writers, Sigurd Olson. He lived from 1899 to 1982, and his passion was the wilderness. He was accused on occasion of finding all civilization and technology "bad," but this was not the case. Sigurd simply treasured the wild places and their power to regenerate spirits, souls, and bodies, and he sought both to preserve them and to usher others into them at every opportunity.

I believe something similar could be said here about those of us who are passionate about natural birth.

Appropriately utilized medicalized birth is indispensable. When medicine isn't required—which we now know is most of the time—the act of giving birth naturally is more than indispensable. It's a transformational, even transcendent event. The chance to experience it must be preserved for those desiring to experience it, and those equipped to usher others into such experiences require preservation, too. (65)

"We're trying to bridge the gap between our old (human) wisdom, our old primeval consciousness, the old verities, and the strange, conflicting ideologies and beliefs of the new era of technology.

One of the most vital tasks of modern man is to bridge this gap... None of us is naïve enough to want to give up what technology has brought or to evade the challenges now before us. This too is a frontier, not only of the mind but of the physical world. Somehow we must make the adjustment and bring both ways of life together. If man can do this, if he can span past and present, then he can face the future with confidence." —Sigurd F. Olson, Conservationist and Activist, *The Meaning of Wilderness* (66)

"There's an irreducible incidence
of complications in human obstetrics…"

Robert Bradley, MD; *Husband-Coached Childbirth*

…

"Birth is as safe as life gets."

a favorite saying among midwives

# 4

# RISK

Kate jotted her findings in Lillian's chart, then sent her assistant, Sarah, a text. "She's doing it! Contractions are 3-4 minutes apart and lasting 70-90 seconds. Gonna set up."

Sarah texted back, "Woohoo! And I'm here."

Bear welcomed Sarah inside, and the two women went to work.

Lillian and John moved to the bathroom to fulfill the classic midwifery recommendation to "have five contractions on the toilet," while Kate and Sarah made up the bed—sheets, plastic, sheets, two under pads, and an inviting pile of pillows. Sarah folded the comforter into a corner of the bedroom while Kate set up the oxygen and accoutrements—Resus-A-Cradle, heating pad, and stack of blue and green receiving blankets into another corner. Lillian had made the blankets herself from an older set of flannel sheets and was very pleased with them.

Kate then drew up an ampule of Pitocin and opened two plastic trash bags. She hung the bags on a door handle, then crouched beside Sarah and the couple's box of supplies.

They opened and folded a prodigious stack of under pads, tore off and folded twenty sheets of paper towel, and filled a squirt bottle with almond oil. Sarah then trotted off to the kitchen with the remainder of the paper towels and the bottles of rubbing alcohol and hydrogen peroxide.

Kate tucked a stack of clean wash cloths beside her tote and tiptoed into the bathroom with her doppler. John was seated on the edge of the tub, still faithfully rubbing Lillian's back.

"How's it going?" Kate whispered.

"So much pressure," Lillian whispered back, "and some bloody goop."

"Good! John, is she drinking her water?"

"She is."

"Even better."

Ca-click, ca-click, ca-click, ca-click, ca-click, ca-click....



. . . . . . .



I don't mean to present this book as a presumptuous assertion that homebirth is absolutely safe.

No doctor, no nurse, no midwife, nor can any specific setting guarantee a family a safe birth. As Dr. Bradley basically states, there's an unavoidable measure of risk associated with childbearing, and that's no matter the place of birth.

What I can say with confidence, however, is that homebirth midwives are committed to providing their utmost to help the families they serve enjoy birthing experiences as without incident as possible, birthing experiences even as miraculously beautiful as possible.

And still, midwives recognize that when disaster strikes, regardless the statistical chance of such a disaster's occurrence, it's a one hundred percent event for the family affected.

I spent a bit of time talking with a woman recently about the tragic loss of a baby in her family. The baby was born in the hospital as planned, and there she died, immersing those who remained behind her in an ocean of sorrow.

The woman had a lot of questions.

Naturally, as I wasn't there, I could only guess at the answers, but as far as I could ascertain, the mother and child were handled appropriately.

The woman wanted to know if a very subtle change in the baby's heart rate through the last weeks of pregnancy might have been a herald of the impending catastrophe.

I said, "Well, I've seen a lot of babies shift to lower heart rates through the last few weeks of pregnancy and, as long as those numbers remain consistently in the 120-160 range with good variability and good movement, it very rarely proves of concern. In fact, I can't actually think of a time in my own practice such an occurrence has proven of concern. But it may have been a harbinger in your case."

Then I explained the heart of what I really want to share.

If we step back from a single case, as absolutely precious as the people comprising any single case are, and we look at pregnancy and birth from a wider angle, most of the time (again and again and again, even fully 80-85% of the time) both will proceed without issue. That means we have to measure the families we serve from the assumption all is well, only working backward to unwell from there when irregularities or departures from normal actually arise.

Yes! We must listen. Yes! We must watch. Yes! We must take careful note of what we hear and see, but because most families surely will carry and birth their babies without experiencing problems, we just have to repel the temptation to, in fear of the pure myriad of complications possible, treat those families as though they're especially likely to present with any of them.

Our nation's 32% cesarean section rate is a perfect example how mainstream American medicine, per just such fear, has been unable to acknowledge and honor the fact most women and babies are able to move through birth without incident when properly supported. This fear-based point of reference drives those within that system to treat the bulk of those they serve as potential problems and the result, ironically, is a dramatic increase in problems—even the very problems they originally feared.

As a homebirth midwife, I strive to keep my eyes and ears open, and to take careful note of what I observe. Thankfully, most of the issues that arise among the families I tend are noticeable from a distance, and I'm able to secure the additional care required to see everyone safely through. It's always nerve-wracking when a family I serve surprises me with an unlooked-for challenge, though again, thankfully, even then I'm generally able to facilitate safe passage.

And yet, it's purely devastating—and I do truly know this—when I'm surprised with a challenge that arises too suddenly and moves too quickly for me to effect salvage.

When I first began the pursuit of my calling, I stumbled across Dr. Robert Bradley's words, "There's an irreducible incidence of complications in human obstetrics…"

They struck a very sobering chord in my young soul, and I had to decide then and there whether I could serve as a midwife with the reality of them echoing through recesses of my psyche.

The day those echoes overtake me and I begin treating my clients as potential problems versus probable victories will be the day I'll need to bring my calling to close.

No one can tell another soul what to do.

No one but that soul will live with the consequences of their choices.

Happily, however, in the case of birth, the odds are in your favor.

"If you don't know your options, you don't have any."

Diana Korte and Roberta Scaer; *A Good Birth, A Safe Birth*

...

"Life is the sum of all our choices."

Albert Camus

# 5

# OPTIONS

The pair returned to the bedroom and Lillian knelt on the floor to lean over the foot of the bed.

Sarah fetched Lillian a steaming bowl of bone broth and handful of grapes. Lillian sipped and munched between her surges, then moaned and swayed through them.

Sarah and Kate sat in the hallway beside the bedroom door and began filling out the paperwork—a labor flow record, the set of birth summaries with a block for the newborn examination, the three pages of birth certificate worksheets, a piece of card stock called "Welcome, Baby" for the baby's footprints and particulars, and an Eldon Card for typing a sample of blood Kate would draw from a vessel in the baby's cord. Lillian was Rh positive, but it was such a simple thing to check that Kate had adopted the habit of typing each of the babies in her care.

Kate went then to listen to the pitter pattering of the baby's heart and returned to scratch the report into Lillian's chart.

"John just texted for Annie to come," Kate whispered to Sarah.

Annie was the woman John and Lillian had invited to care for Sawyer, their older child, through the birth. They wanted him present if all was going well.

"I love it when birth is a family event," Sarah said.

"I do, too." Kate smiled as she cracked open her thermos of coffee.

. . . . . . .

Without accurate knowledge, provided without bias—or possibly simply with bias attribution—however can we hope to make solid decisions?

## Informed Disclosure

Homebirth midwifery care is a wonderful series of friendly visits that begin with a meeting where a family is able to assess a person's potential to serve well as their midwife, and where that midwife is able to assess a family regarding their homebirth eligibility. The meeting usually begins with all sorts of questions and includes a description of the midwife's education and experience, a listing of her statistics— adverse outcomes included—and copies of her policies, practice guidelines, and informed disclosure statements.

After that initial gathering, the family spends some time considering if that particular midwife is the right fit for them. If she is the right fit and, of course, if the family is eligible for a homebirth, then commences a relationship that, professionally, will span from seven to eight months and, personally, will likely last a lifetime.

The next step for the midwife to make is that of making sure the expectant family is making a fully informed decision regarding their desire to birth at home.

Here's part of what I share with folks who think they want to birth their babies at home with me.

I read a beautiful book recently, *When Breath Becomes Air*, by Paul Kalanithi, MD. (67) In it he describes awakening to a clearer view of informed consent—something fuller, something richer than simply listing potential hazards, clarifying limitations, assigning expectations and responsibilities, and signing along dotted lines. Paul woke to see the process of obtaining informed consent more the forging of a covenant between souls. An offering to walk with another as she seeks to navigate a portion of the hills and valleys of her existence.

That resonated with me.

To paraphrase Paul's words: Yes, if you decide you want to join hands with me as you plunge into the adventure of parenthood, there will be specific things we'll expect from each other, a listing of responsibilities as well as acknowledgements of limitations and etcetera, but in the midst of that, it's very simply this—I've been where you're going. I know the way. I'm merely a mortal, so I can't foresee the future or promise an outcome, but I can offer you the benefit of my experience, my knowledge, my skill, my intuition, and the fact that I care about you. If you choose to take my hand, I'll guide you to the best of my abilities as we walk together through the twists and dips and turns—I'll walk with you until we make it to the other side.

The midwifery relationship is one founded on trust. I expect honesty from the families I serve and they can expect the same from me.

I believe it's your right to be fully responsible for your health care. If you hire me, I'll provide examination, assessment, information, and advice regarding all aspects of your pregnancy, childbearing, new parenting, and post-birth recovery in order to help you enjoy the outcome you desire. These services and resources will be provided primarily through our prenatal appointments, through my attendance of your labor and birth, and through our postpartum visits.

The period of time spanning both the approach and the arrival of a new baby is both a very special one *and* a very challenging one. Please ask every question you have, and ask on until you understand the answers you receive. If you're not satisfied with my answers, let me know. And please don't hesitate to contact me if you need additional help. I'm more than willing to make extra visits to assist you during this vulnerable stage of your life. If I'm unable to provide the aid you require, I'll make every effort to put you in touch with someone who can.

I understand you and I will not always see every facet of your health and care the same way. I fully recognize that your health and care are, indeed, yours, and I stand ready to accept and respect your decisions.

Similarly, an aspect of the care I provide is the desire to complete care of a family with a healthy midwife as well as with a healthy mom and baby. The quote, "A healthy mom and healthy baby," has been restated within the midwifery community as, "safe for the mom, safe for the baby, safe for the midwife." While all midwives may be created equal, not all midwives are equally suited to all tasks. Based on an infinite and ever-changing array of variables arising out of her unique mix of training, knowledge, experience, and level of comfort, each midwife must determine for herself whether she's the best provider of care for the client at hand. In other words, there will inevitably be times when I'll feel obligated to discontinue care of a client simply because I'm not, or perceive that I'm not, as described above, equal to the task.

When "safe for the mom, safe for the baby, safe for the midwife" makes it necessary to discontinue care of a client, I provide my reasons in written form, as well as at a visit in person. I also do my utmost to assist the client in her efforts to secure the services of other, more appropriate care.

One essential component of this is your commitment to fully utilize the services I provide. Please let me know if there are any obstacles to your ability to utilize my services.

Whomever you invite to serve you as you move through this pinnacle of human events, make sure you receive something similar to what I've shared here in this chapter, and even here in this book. It's of prime importance you know exactly who your provider is—their education, their level of experience, their track-record, their philosophy, and their level of commitment to you and your needs and desires.

The same should be sought from the facility you intend to employ, if you elect to birth away from home.

"Again, the obvious ego-deflating question was put to me
as the obstetrician: "Who needs a doctor for this?"

Robert Bradley, MD; *Husband-Coached Childbirth* (44)

. . .

"Changes in birthing practices that allow women
to rediscover the spontaneous sexual rhythms of labor
are not, by and large, coming from within obstetrics.
They're coming from pressure by women to have
the chance to birth in their own way, in their own
time, in an emotionally supportive setting,
and with uninhibited and joyous birth passion."

Sheila Kitzinger; from the forward to
Dr. Odent's *Birth Reborn* (4)

"If we hope to create a world where respect and kindness replace fear and hatred, we must begin by how we treat each other at the beginning of life, for that is where our deepest patterns are set. From these roots grow fear and alienation or love and trust."

Suzanne Arms; *Immaculate Deception* (68)

...

"The idea of some sort of medication being utilized in such an efficient, peaceful performance never occurred to the performers and seemed ludicrous to the observers. The close relationship between husband and wife, the total dependence upon each other, was heartwarming to see. That it truly 'takes two to tango' was never more manifest."

Robert Bradley, MD; *Husband-Coached Childbirth* (44)

# 6

# POSSIBILITIES

Annie arrived just as Kate was returning to the hallway from another heart tone check. She smiled, visibly excited as she settled onto the floor beside the women. Bear flopped down on the floor beside her, laying his big, graying head in her lap as his tail slapped the floor.

Whispers, whispers, whispers.

"How's it going?"

"It's going great! I just sent them back to the bathroom for another five contractions. Sarah, will you run to the kitchen and make up a couple smoothies? John needs to get something in him, and Lillian's finished her broth and her grapes."

"Oh! I can do that!" Annie said.

The smoothies were welcomed by both and, as the trio of ladies listened from the other side of the doors, they noticed with pleasure as

Lillian's rushes became ever stronger and closer and more intense.

After one especially long and strong wave Lillian said, "Ugh. I feel like I might get sick."

Kate and Sarah sprang to their feet. Sarah snatched up one of the washcloths from beside the tote and ran it under a stream of cold water while Kate opened a bottle of peppermint oil under Lillian's nose.

"Take a good sniff of this, Lillian," Kate said, and Sarah draped the cool cloth across the nape of her neck.

"I feel like I can't do this anymore," Lillian whimpered with a trash can fairly crushed between her knees.

"That's a really good sign," Kate said, "and you're doing so, so well."

A shudder swept Lillian's frame, making her teeth chatter.

"Are you su—sure?"

"I'm sure."

"She's sure," John echoed, "and you're amazing."

. . . . . . .

For many, once the question of safety is adequately answered— once they understand most low-risk moms will be able to birth their low-risk babies without issue—they're left with the realization they can experience their birth however they want to experience their birth.

Your journey into parenthood began when you fell in love with your life partner, when you made love with your life partner, when your lovemaking created a new life.

The conditions best for entering into parenthood—for birthing—are very much the same as those that got you started.

Giving birth is your love come full circle.

When it comes down to it, just be ready to do what you do when you make love. Carve out a beautiful space. Fill it with music and soft sheets and lovely scents. Dim the lights and light the candles. Close the door. Cling to one another. Remember that making love is a thing you surrender to, a thing that both schools you and unleashes you as it sweeps you along.

Let go as the sensations build and follow your instincts. Moan and writhe and cry out—do all and whatever you must to reach your climax.

Then drop back upon the pillows and bask in the glow—this time with a warm, wet, wriggling mass of life pressed against your heaving breasts.

If birth needn't be a medical event, it may simply be a life event—a family event.

And so, yes—once the question of safety is adequately answered, all that remains is the question—what exactly are you wanting for your birthing experience?

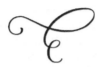

"The best way out is always through."

Robert Frost, "A Servant to Servants"

...

"...Come... sense the sacredness of all creation."

David Backes, from the introduction to Sigurd Olson's
*The Meaning of Wilderness* (66)

# 7

# SACRED

Lillian moved from the toilet and climbed to her hands and knees on the bed. John scrambled up beside her just as another powerful wave rose and swept her quaking form.

She breathed and breathed, then arched her back slightly.

"Ooooooohhh—ooh—ahhhhh…."

Sarah and Kate looked at each other and raised their eyebrows.

"Annie," Kate whispered, "why don't you go get Sawyer."

"Is it time already?" she whispered back.

"I think so."

Sarah and Kate knelt on the floor beside the bed. Annie brought Sawyer in from his room toasty-warm, tousle-headed, sleepy-eyed, and settled onto a chair under the window.

"Baby?" he said to Annie.

"Soon."

He snuggled into her lap and popped a stubby thumb into his

mouth.

Another great wave began to swell and Lillian said, "Oh my gosh! I think I'm pushing! Aahhhgggggrrrrrrr—rrrgohh—oh, oh—aahhh...."

"Okay, Lillian, easy now. Let's just keep him coming so gentle," Kate said as she reached for her doppler.

Ca-click! Ca-click! Ca-click! Ca-click! Ca-click! Ca-click! Ca-click!

"One fifties. Is the baby moving?"

"He's kicking around like mad!"

The surge began to subside, and the baby's heart rate returned to the one-thirties.

One after another, potent, almost insistent waves rolled and broke over Lillian. Sometimes she grunted, sometimes she groaned, always and forever she breathed.

A ribbon of glowing sky brightened the room and a shimmering, fluid-filled oval appeared from the folds of Lillian's womanhood.

A breath. A groan.

A robin called out.

Ca-click, ca-click....

A breath.

A breeze rustled the curtains and a sparkling shaft of gold parted the layers of clouds lining the horizon.

A breath. A groan. A grunt. A gasp. A breath.

The shimmering oval expanded.

A breath.

Ca-click, ca-click, ca-click, ca-click....

A second robin called.

A breath. A breath. A catch. A grunt.

"Aaahhhhhhh!"

A small, round head pressed itself past Lillian's spreading flesh,

98

still enclosed in that shimmering, translucent oval of tissue. Flecks of creamy white vernix floated in the waters over a fine lace work of violet veins and sandy strands of hair.

John shifted to Lillian's feet, his hand stretching toward all that glistened as a tear trickled the length of his nose.

Poousshhh....

Drip....

Plish... plish....

A perfect face turned slowly toward John.

John gingerly peeled filaments of sac from the wee mouth and nose.

A breath. A breath. A breath. A grunt.

The child traced a graceful arc as he spun into his father's hands, and a fiery ball of sun gushed into a radiant sky!

"Oh!" his mother said.

"Oh!" said his father as he began to sob, "Oh, honey, you did it!"

A whole assembly of robins erupted into torrents of song!

And a brand-new life set the air ringing with an ever-strengthening wail!

Lillian turned herself over and extended her arms, and John laid their son in them, bursting into second freshet of tears as he did.

Annie set Sawyer on the bed and he scooted his diapered bottom till he was cuddled up at mom's side and, with his thumb still stashed amidst his lips, he wondered over his little brother.

"Baby?" he asked with wide, unblinking eyes.

"Yes, Sweetie," his mama said, "this is the baby."

"Hey, Baby."

"Yeah," John said. "Hey, Baby."

Through the next couple hours Lillian brought her placenta forth, the baby kicked and wiggled himself onto his mother's breast, and the family had a meal of oatmeal and eggs as the women charted and tidied the room—all seven basking in the glorious afterglow of Cedar's birth.

Lillian was thrilled to learn her netherlands were intact and, after John and Sawyer severed Cedar's cord, the newborn examination was enjoyed by all—seemingly even by Cedar who gazed as intently at Kate as she gazed intently at him.

That evening Kate received a text from Lillian.

"So—here I am, out on the deck with John. Sawyer, who couldn't stop saying, 'the baby came OUT!' all day, finally fell asleep. My feet are up, Cedar's at my breast, and I'm having a glass of wine while the sun sets and the robins sing their goodnight melodies to us. Kate, when I said I loved my hospital birth and wasn't the homebirthing type—well, I just didn't know. I don't know how many other babies I'll have, but I'll never go back. I'm a believer."

. . . . . . .

Currently a mere percent of American moms give birth to their babies at home, but of those who do, most would "never go back" to the hospital.

I hope this book has shown you that most women could very safely and very happily birth their babies in their homes should they so desire and need "never go back."

Maybe you're one of them.

# REFERENCES

1. **Leboyer, F.** *Birth without violence.* London : Pinter and Martin, 2011.

2. **McDonald, L.** *Birth Journeys: Positive birth stories to encourage and inspire.* EBook : Star Class, 2012.

3. **Macari, M.** *She Births.* PA : Infinity Publishing, 2014.

4. **Odent, M.** *Birth Reborn: What Childbirth Should Be.* London : Souvenir Press Ltd, 1994.

5. **Frye, A.** *Holistic Midwifery Volume II.* OR : Labrys, 2013.

6. **Cheyney M, Bovbjerg M, Everson C et al.** Outcomes of Care for 16,924 Planned Home Births in the United States: The Midwives Alliance of North America Statistics Project, 2004 to 2009. *Journal of Midwifery and Women's Health.* 59(1): 17-27, 2014.

7. **Wax JR, Lucus FL, Lamont M.** Maternal and Newborn Outcomes in Planned Home Birth vs Planned Hospital Birth: A Meta-analysis. *American Journal of Obstetrics and Gynecology.* 203(3):243.e1-8, 2010.

8. **Michal C, Janssen P, Vedam S et al.** Planned Home vs. Hospital Birth: A Meta–Analysis Gone Wrong. *Medscape .* [Online] 2011. https://www.medscape.com/viewarticle/739987.

9. **Moore, J.** Why Not Home? The Surprising Birth Choices of Doctors and *Nurses.* [Video] 2016.

10. **Brocklehurst P, Hardy P, Hollowell J et al.** Perinatal and maternal outcomes by planned place of birth for healthy women with low risk pregnancies: the Birthplace in England national prospective cohort study. *British Medical Journal.* 343:d7400, 2011.

11. **Homer CS, Thornton C, Scarf VL et al.** Birthplace in New South Wales, Australia: an analysis of perinatal outcomes using routinely collected data. *BMC Pregnancy & Childbirth.* 14:206, 2014.

12. **de Jonge A, Geerts CC, van der Goes BY et al.** Perinatal mortality and morbidity up to 28 days after birth among 743 070 low-risk planned home and hospital births: a cohort study based on three merged national perinatal databases. *British Journal of Obstetrics and Gynaecology.* 122(5):720-8, 2015.

13. **Scarf VL, Rossiter C, Vedam S et al.** Maternal and perinatal outcomes by planned place of birth among women with low-risk pregnancies in high-income countries: A systematic review and meta-analysis. *Midwifery.* 62:240-255, 2018.

14. **Hutton EK, Reitsma A, Simioni J et al.** Perinatal or neonatal mortality among women who intend at the onset of labour to give birth at home compared to women of low obstetrical risk who intend to give birth in hospital: A systematic review and meta-analyses. *The Lancet.* doi.org/10.1016/j.eclinm.2019.07.005, 2019.

15. **Goer, H.** Research Review: Systematic Review Finds No Increase in Adverse Outcomes with Planned Home Birth. *Connecting the Dots.* [Online] https://www.lamaze.org/Connecting-the-Dots/Post/research-review-systematic-review-finds-no-increase-in-adverse-outcomes-with-planned-home-birth-1.

16. **North American Registry of Midwives.** *(NARM).* [Online] https://narm.org/about-narm/.

17. **Daviss, B-A, Johnson K.** Outcomes of Planned Home Births with Certified Professional Midwives: Large Prospective Study in North America. *British Medical Journal.* 330:1416, 2005.

18. **Martin, N.** A Larger Role for Midwives Could Improve Deficient U.S. Care for Mothers and Babies. *ProPublica.* [Online] 2018. https://www.propublica.org/article/midwives-study-maternal-neonatal-care.

19. **de Jonge A, Van der Goes B, Ravelli A.** Perinatal Mortality and Morbidity in a Nationwide Cohort of 529,688 Low-Risk Planned Home and Hospital Births. *British Journal of Obstetrics and Gynaecology.* 116(9):1177-84, 2009.

20. **Wagner, M.** Fish Can't See Water: The Need to Humanize Birth. *International Journal of Gynaecology and Obstetrics.* 75 Suppl 1:S25-37, 2001.

21. —. Technology in Birth: First Do No Harm. *Midwifery Today.* [Online] 2000. https://midwiferytoday.com/web-article/technology-birth-first-no-harm/.

22. **Heubeck, E.** Midwives Could Be Key in Reversing Maternal Mortality Trends. *Connecticut Health I-Team.* [Online] 2018. http://c-hit.org/2018/10/30/midwives-could-be-key-to-reversing-maternal-mortality-trends/.

23. **Midwives Alliance North America.** The Midwives Model of Care. *(MANA).* [Online] 2016. https://mana.org/about-midwives/midwifery-model.

24. **American Academy of Pediatrics.** Conflicts between Religious or Spiritual Beliefs and Pediatric Care: Informed Refusal, Exemptions, and Public Funding. *Pediatrics.* 132:5, 2013.

25. **Center for Poverty Research.** How is poverty related to access to care and preventive healthcare? [Online] 2015. https://poverty.ucdavis.edu/faq/how-poverty-related-access-care-and-preventive-healthcare.

26. **Villarosa, L.** America's Black Mothers and Babies are in a Life-or-Death Crisis. *The New York Times.* [Online] https://www.nytimes.com/2018/04/11/magazine/black-mothers-babies-death-maternal-mortality.html.

27. **Wickham, S.** Birthillogics #1 – Induction for Advanced Maternal Age. *www.sarawickham.com.* [Online] https://www.sarawickham.com/birthillogics/birthillogics-1-induction-for-advanced-maternal-age/.

28. —. Birth outcomes and women of size. *www.sarawickham.com.* [Online] 2015. https://www.sarawickham.com/research-updates/birth-outcomes-and-women-of-size/.

29. **National LGBT Health Education Center.** Understanding the Health Needs of LGBT People. [Online] 2016. https://www.lgbthealtheducation.org/wp-content/uploads/LGBTHealthDisparitiesMar2016.pdf.

30. **Grobman WA, Bailit JL, Rice MM.** Racial and ethnic disparities in maternal morbidity and obstetric care. *Obstetrics and Gynecology.* 125(6):1460-7, 2015.

31. **Darling EK, Lawford KMO, Wilson K et al.** Distance from Home Birth to Emergency Obstetric Services and Neonatal Outcomes: A Cohort Study. *Journal of Midwifery and Women's Health.* 64(2):170-178, 2019.

32. **Davis, E.** *Orgasmic Birth: Your Guide to a Safe, Satisfying, and Pleasurable Birth Experience.* PA : Rodale Publishing, 2010.

33. **Gaskin, IM.** *Ina May's Guide to Childbirth.* NY : Bantam Dell, 2003.

34. **Lothian, J.** Saying "No" to Induction. *The Journal of Perinatal Education.* 15(2): 43–45, 2006.

35. **Wickham, S.** *Inducing Labour: making informed decisions.* Avebury : Birthmoon Creations, 2018.

36. **Morley, G.** Neonatal Resuscitation: Life that Failed. *OB-GYN.net.* [Online] 2003. https://www.obgyn.net/articles/neonatal-resuscitation-life-failed.

37. **Edwards N, Wickham S.** *Birthing Your Placenta: the third stage of labour.* Avebury : Birthmoon Creations, 2018.

38. **Kangaroo Mother Care.** Fathers and Skin-to-Skin Contact. *Kangaroo Mother Care.* [Online] 2018. https://kangaroomothercare.com/about-kmc/fathers-and-skin-to-skin-contact/.

39. —. For Full Term Babies . *Kangaroo Mother Care.* [Online] 2018. http://www.kangaroomothercare.com/about-kmc/for-full-term-babies/.

40. **Bergman, J.** The Importance of Skin to Skin Contact for Every Newborn. *Kangaroo Mother Care.* [Online] 2011. http://kangaroomothercare.com/articles/jills-articles/.

41. **Olanders, M.** Kangaroo Mother Care: An Interview with Dr. Nils Bergman. *Primal Page.* [Online] 2011. http://www.primal-page.com/eng-berg.html.

42. **Kangaroo Mother Care.** Separation and Stress. *Kangaroo Mother Care.* [Online] 2018. http://www.kangaroomothercare.com/about-kmc/separation-and-stress/.

43. **Margulis, J.** What if Homebirth is Actually SAFER than Hospital Birth? *reset.me.* [Online] 2016. https://reset.me/story/what-if-home-birth-is-actually-safer-than-hospital-birth/.

44. **Bradley, R.** *Husband-coached Childbirth: The Bradley Method of Natural Childbirth* . NY : Bantam, 2008.

45. **Maternal Health Task Force.** Maternal Health in the United States. *Maternal Health Task Force.* [Online] 2019. https://www.mhtf.org/topics/maternal-health-in-the-united-states/.

46. **Moriarty, E.** Maternal Mortality: An American Crisis. *CBS News.* [Online] 2018. https://www.cbsnews.com/news/maternal-mortality-an-american-crisis/.

47. **Martin N, Montague R.** U.S. Has the Worst Rate of Maternal Deaths in the Developed World. *NPR News.* [Online] https://www.npr.org/2017/05/12/528098789/u-s-has-the-worst-rate-of-maternal-deaths-in-the-developed-world.

48. **Gonzales S, Sawyer B.** How Does Infant Mortality in the U.S. Compare to Other Countries? *Peterson-Kaiser Health System Tracker.* [Online] 2017. https://www.healthsystemtracker.org/chart-collection/infant-mortality-u-s-compare-countries.

49. **Gregory KD, Jackson S, Korst L et al.** Cesarean versus vaginal delivery: whose risks? Whose benefits? *American Journal of Perinatology.* 29(1):7-18, 2012.

50. **Molina G, Weiser TG, Lipsitz SR et al.** Relationship Between Cesarean Delivery Rate and Maternal and Neonatal Mortality. *Journal of the American Medical Association.* 314(21):2263-70, 2015.

51. **The Leapfrog Group.** Rate of C-Sections. *Leapfrog.* [Online] 2018. https://www.leapfroggroup.org/ratings-reports/rate-c-sections.

52. **Sandall J, Soltani H, Gates S et al.** Midwife-led continuity models versus other models of care for childbearing women. *Cochrane Database of Systematic Reviews.* Issue 4. Art. No.: CD004667. DOI: 10.1002/14651858.CD004667.pub5, 2016.

53. **Centers for Disease Control and Prevention.** Severe Maternal Morbidity in the United States. *Centers for Disease Control and Prevention.* [Online] 2016. https://www.cdc.gov/reproductivehealth/maternalinfanthealth/severe maternalmorbidity.html.

54. **The Mayo Clinic.** Forceps Delivery. *Mayo Clinic.* [Online] 2018. https://www.mayoclinic.org/tests-procedures/forceps-delivery/about/pac-20394207.

55. —. C Section. *Mayo Clinic.* [Online] 2018. https://www.mayoclinic.org/tests-procedures/c-section/about/pac-20393655.

56. **Jansen L, Gibson M, Bowles B et al.** First Do No Harm: Interventions During Childbirth. *The Journal of Perinatal Education.* 22(2): 83–92, 2013.

57. **Curtin SC, Gregory KD, Korst LM et al.** Maternal Morbidity for Vaginal and Cesarean Deliveries According to Previous Cesarean History: New Data from the Birth Certificate, 2013. *National Vital Statistics Reports.* 64(4):1-13, 2015.

58. **Buckley, S.** Hormonal Physiology of Childbearing: Evidence and Implications for Women, Babies, and Maternity Care. *Journal of Perinatal*

*Education.* 24(3): 145–153, 2015.

59. **Uvnäs-Moberg K, Ekström-Bergström A, Berg M et al.**
Maternal plasma levels of oxytocin during physiological childbirth – a systematic review with implications for uterine contractions and central actions of oxytocin. *BMC Pregnancy and Childbirth.* 19: 285, 2019.

60. **Wickham, S.** Oxytocin and Birth: the latest evidence. *www.sarawickham.com.* [Online] 2019. https://www.sarawickham.com/research-updates/oxytocin-and-birth-the-latest-evidence/.

61. **Buckley, S.** Epidurals: Risks and Concerns for Mother and Baby. [Online] 2018. https://www.mhtf.org/topics/maternal-health-in-the-united-states/.

62. **The Mayo Clinic.** Vacuum Extraction. *Mayo Clinic.* [Online] 2018. https://www.mayoclinic.org/tests-procedures/vacuum-extraction/about/pac-20395232.

63. **Shorten, A.** Maternal and Neonatal Effects of Caesarean Section. *British Medical Journal.* 335:1003, 2007.

64. **Dunn AB, Jordan S, Baker BJ.** The Maternal Infant Microbiome: Considerations for Labor and Birth. *MCN: American Journal of Maternal-Child Nursing.* 42(6): 318–325, 2018.

65. **Kline, W.** To Lower Maternal and Infant Mortality Rates, We Need More Midwives. *The Washington Post.* [Online] 2019. https://www.washingtonpost.com/outlook/2019/01/16/lower-maternal-infant-mortality-rates-we-must-bring-back-midwives.

66. **Olsen, SF.** *The Meaning of Wilderness.* Minneapolis : University of Minnesota Press, 2015.

67. **Kalanithi, P.** *When Breath Becomes Air.* New York : Vintage, 2017.

68. **Arms, S.** *Immaculate Deception.* Boston : Houghton Mifflin, 1975.

"Rather than love, than money, than fame, give me truth."

Henry David Thoreau

…

"Whenever you find yourself on the side of the majority,
it's time to pause and reflect."

Mark Twain

…

"The way we do anything is the way we do everything."

Martha Beck, "The Labyrinth of Life"

# ACKNOWLEDGEMENTS

Though I've striven only to share facts in this book, I realize what I've shared stands to be hard for the thousands of American medical personnel serving the multiplying element of our population to read.

I realize what I've shared stands to hurt them and even possibly to anger them.

That's far from my heart.

I realize, too, and without a doubt, however what I've written may affect our nation's hardworking medical personnel, it's been hardest for the families who've experienced childbirth-related losses—from death to damage to dissatisfactory experiences—the families, the people who represent the facts shared in this little book—to suffer those losses and then to try to live with those losses.

To those families, I acknowledge your losses.

We all do—I just know we do—and I know we all grieve with you, too.

My hope is this little book will cause pause, will stimulate thought, will inspire assessment and reassessment.

My hope is this little book will be another log on the fire of change.

So many priceless lives depend on it.

And many, many, many thanks to Steven Osterholzer, my beloved husband. Without you and your indescribable support and your actual physical help—provided, no less, while away on our vacation—it literally would not exist.

And many, many, many, many, many—oh! Even numberless thank yous to my friend, Dr. Sara Wickham!

I mailed this book in as finished a form as I was able to muster, hoping and praying she'd read it, like it, and endorse it.

She did me one better. She began by suggesting we reformat the references, then suggested we strengthen my positions with additional references, and then suggested I add "Commonly Asked Questions" — something I originally wrote as a separate piece—as an appendix.

I won't lie. I was daunted by her suggestions. I asked almost whimsically if she'd like to implement them herself. I nearly fainted when she said, "Yes!"

Less than forty-eight hours later, this beautifully improved version of the book arrived in my inbox, and warm, salty tears sprang into my eyes.

# COMMONLY ASKED QUESTIONS

## Is it expensive?

Compared to birth in the hospital, homebirth midwifery is inexpensive indeed.

The range of homebirth midwifery fees vary widely from state to state, and even from county to county within each state. The primary factor contributing to the cost of homebirth midwifery services is generally the region's cost of living index.

Commonly the price of a homebirth midwife is equal to or even a bit less than insurance deductibles for hospital births.

## Will my insurance cover it?

Increasingly, measures of insurance reimbursement are made available to homebirth midwives, though it still tends to be a seriously crazy endeavor where only those who handle the claims just exactly so manage to receive a check.

To maximize our chances of success, many of us hire midwifery-oriented insurance billing agencies to file our clients' claims.

## Is it messy?

Birth certainly bears the potential to be messy but, between the list of items your midwife will have you purchase in anticipation of your birth, your midwife's mad skills at using those items, and the fact that should there be an item or item-handler malfunction of some sort your midwife will have an extra set of chores to accomplish before she can go home, the chance you or your belongings will suffer damage through the experience of your birth is slight.

A goal of most midwives is to leave you, yours, and your home with the baby as the only tangible evidence the birth ever occurred.

## What about the pain?

Sadly, our culture has so thoroughly conditioned women to believe we're unequal to the aim of birthing our babies without pain palliation, many if not most of us plan to proceed within arm's reach of an anesthesiologist.

This hurts my heart.

Your body was literally designed to give birth to your babies.

Every sensation you experience while working to give birth to your baby is generated by your own body.

The sensations you experience while working with your body's incredible and innate baby-birthing design comprise the release of a delicious mix of hormones, a series of stunning alterations, an utterly astounding display of power, and one of the very most poignant moments of your entire life.

What, then of pain?

Waves…. Rushes…. Surges…. Sensations….

Transformation.

Pain….

Metamorphosis.

This process occurs most effectively when it proceeds in private, within an abundance of loving and respectful support, and minus unnecessary fiddling.

When the process proceeds in private, within an abundance of loving and respectful support, and minus unnecessary fiddling, pain is experienced, but scarcely does it become an issue.

Again.

Your body was literally designed to give birth to your babies.

Every sensation you experience while working to give birth to your baby is generated by your own body.

Again.

Your journey into parenthood began when you fell in love with your life partner, when you made love with your life partner, when your lovemaking created a new life.

The conditions best for making the plunge into parenthood—for birthing—are very much the same as those that got you started.

Again.

It's your love come full circle.

Women who birth at home—surrounded by privacy, by love and respect, by peace, and by quiet—choose to embrace the pain.

And they find they're equal to it.

## Can my husband and/or children participate?

When birth proceeds according to its incredible, innate design, the most appropriate thing is for husbands and children to join mothers and babies as the central participants—for, indeed, if birth needn't be a medical event, it may simply be a family event.

Midwives love witnessing little ones emerge into the light as their fathomless eyes wink and peek beneath downy brows, but what many midwives love best is when this transpires under and into the strong, yet gentle hands of fathers, with the rest of the family gathered at his elbows in awestruck wonder.

Through the inimitable process of natural and unmedicated childbirth, oxytocin, the "fall-in-love" hormone, and endorphins, the hormones of pain alleviation, flood and gush through the veins of mother and baby, transporting both into altered states of consciousness. Incredibly, when a man, the lover of that woman and the father of that baby, intimately experiences the exquisite pain and poignancy of birth, equal measures of "fall-in-love" hormone suffuse his own veins with every pulsating thrum of his heart.

When this man, with every morsel of his being awash and alive in that brew of tender devotion, spreads his hands to receive his tiny child, that burgeoning life, that fruit of his ardor and passion emerging from the secret places of his beloved, he pauses… one heartbeat… two heartbeats… three… suspended in the holiness of the moment until he draws in a great shuddering breath and exhales, "Oh! Ooooohh!! Oooooooohhh!!!"

Then, hovering there over those two souls, more precious to him than life itself, he bursts into tears.

Midwives sit just off to the side, assessing mom and baby with their eyes and ears, with their knowledge and experience and common sense, discreetly hemming in the mess and reveling in the enchantment as they watch and wait to be needed.

The woman lies in quietness a moment before gathering herself to greet her child. The child lies in the grip of his father's hands, little arms and legs spread wide, spluttering and dribbling as he fills the world with his cries. The man, still exulting and exclaiming, praising his love in

116

sob-clotted gushes, tears streaming from his cheeks and trickling from the tip of his nose, gingerly places the wailing baby upon his wife's sweaty breasts while those tears splash all over them... as though watering them....

As though baptizing them.

Not every daddy is able to catch his own baby. Some mothers desire to receive the child with their own hands, or sometimes a mama hops into some unexpected position that puts her husband's hands out of reach, or very possibly her sinewy arms will be wrapped so snug around her man's neck that to loose himself would be to disturb her. Sometimes a baby needs a little help in his effort to slide earthside, enough help, such help, as the midwife winds up with him in her own hands. And some dads would just really rather not do the actual catching.

Yet whomever receives the baby, when that baby does at last arrive, encircled by father and siblings as they hold their breath—

As they shed their tears—

As they erupt with pure joy—

Oh! Would that we all be so welcomed into our lives!

What sort of difference would that make in our world, I wonder?

# AND FINALLY

*"I've been chided for my penchant for posting 'baby' every time I attend a birth and I've been questioned as to the appropriateness of sharing birth photographs and films in public as well, but as long as so much misinformation and misunderstanding regarding homebirth exists—especially among the medical community and especially the way this misinformation and misunderstanding threatens families' freedom to pursue homebirth as an option—I'll be sharing these pictures and films every chance I get, and I'll be posting 'baby' after every single birth I attend."*

I shared this on Facebook in 2019 in the context of a conversation I'd had with a hospital-based birthworker about homebirth transfers.

A month or so later, I was discussing all this with my son—my homeborn son and the father of two of my homeborn grandbabies.

He fetched a calculator.

"How many babies are born at home in the US every year, Mom?"

I told him one percent of four million.

"Okay," he said, tapping away at the little keys, "that's 40,000 homebirths a year... 3,333 births a month and..."

Tap, tap, tap...

"about 109 births per day."

I was stunned.

And then he suggested we—all of us homebirth midwives—use the hashtag #birthsafeathome with something like "Baby!" every time we usher another new little one into life at home in order to create a universally accessible database demonstrating just how very much more often homebirth is truly safe than otherwise.

Friends, let's do this! Let's really show the world who we are and what we do!

What do you say?

I say, "Baby!"

#birthsafeathome
#homebirthsafeandsacred

Made in the USA
Middletown, DE
26 February 2022

61826742R00070